How to Get Your Child to Succeed in Life

DEAN KIM

ISBN:
ISBN-13: 978-1975806309
ISBN-10:1975806301

DEDICATION

To my father who taught me all about life and being the best father anyone could ever hope for…Thank you for everything, your guidance, wisdom and always being my pillar of strength.

CONTENTS

ACKNOWLEDGMENTS

I'd like to acknowledge and thank the following people for my inspiration in writing this book. Thank you, Master Melody Shuman who has influenced me on teaching young children since the 1990's. I have learned so much from you over the years and continue to do so. Thank you, Team Parrella for showing me the technical know how and motivation to write this book. And of course I like to thank my students. I learned from all of you over the years as well as teaching you martial arts over the years. It is great to know so many wonderful people can impact our community and the world in such a positive way. You make me proud as an instructor, a master, but most importantly as a person because knowing all of you has enriched my life.

1
PREFACE

What are the martial arts? Most people think of fighting, kicking, punching, Mixed Martial Arts, Ultimate Fighting Championship, Jackie Chan and Jet Li movies.

Martial arts has a small part of "fighting", specifically self-defense. We train to "fight" so we don't have to fight.

The Martial arts are about respect. Respect for one's self, people, and all living things. The Martial arts develops in people - confidence, focus, concentration, discipline, self-esteem, courage, integrity, balance, coordination, honor, loyalty, humility, patience, setting and achieving goals, and personal growth development. Martial arts reinforce a person's value system. In short it is philosophy, not a cult, nor is it a religion.

A martial artist does improve a person's physical fitness level. Everyone starts at some level and with training can improve their level over time.

Doctor's always recommend eating healthy, exercise, and get the proper amount of rest. The Martial Arts are a great way to exercise and learn self-defense along the way.

2
INTRODUCTION

You want the best for your child. You want the best education for your child, the best childhood, having your kid be the leader of his/her group of friends, not a follower. As a parent, you will do anything to make sure your child is successful.

So, in today's busy times, how as a parent do you do that? You can not be with him or her twenty-four seven. You worry about what if he gets in with the wrong crowd, what if he can't make friends, what is influencing your child, who are his role models, what if this happens or what if that happens, what if, what if, what if?

You heard karate creates discipline for children, but where do you go, what do you look for? What kind of karate should he or she take, which one is best for kids, how do you know it will work? Will he listen to the teacher if he doesn't always listen to you?

You want your kid to be better, physically, mentally, emotionally and socially. Martial art does exactly this. So, when do you have your kid start martial arts? 4 years old? 7? 10?

Here at Karate Universe we take children as soon as they are potty trained and here is why. Young children are naturally learning and every experience is new for them. They are a blank slate and can learn good habits right from the start. Little kids little problems, big kids big problems. It is easier to get a young child to listen to you and get in the habit of doing the right thing than a 16 or 17-year-old that is six feet four and tells you he's taking the car and there is not a damn thing you can do about it. Respect has to be instilled at a young age. Children need to learn to respect their parents, teachers, elders, brothers and sisters, friends and most importantly themselves.

Of course, you want your child to have fun in the process and they do. The "games" we "play" are designed to improve your child's focus, concentration, balance, being able to take turns, socializing and getting along with all kinds of children, learning how to win as well as how to lose. They get physically fit and confident in the process. They get rewarded for doing the right thing. They learn to set goals and achieve them no matter how hard it may seem or how frustrating it can become. They have instructors who want them to succeed and become better and better and guide them through the times when it seems impossible or just plain too hard because they also have been there as well. By sticking with it they learn to persevere and never give up. They do not become aggressive or becoming a bully by training in martial arts. In fact, just the opposite, they stand up to bullies not only for themselves but for their friends as well. They help the weaker kids because they know it is the right thing to do. So how does this all happen? Let's start slow and show you how our students become successful in life.

3

LET'S BEGIN

When do kids start Karate?

As we stated in the introduction, here at Karate Universe we take children as soon as they are potty trained and here is why. Young children are naturally learning and every experience is new for them. They are a blank slate and can learn good habits right from the start. Little kids little problems, big kids big problems. It is easier to get a young child to listen to you and get in the habit of doing the right thing than a 16 or 17-year-old that is six feet four weighs 240 pounds and tells you he's taking the car and there is not a damn thing you can do about it. Respect has to be instilled at a young age. Children need to learn to respect their parents, teachers, elders, brothers and sisters, friends and most importantly themselves.

Every child is different. Some are super shy, some are super aggressive and there is no one teaching method fits all approach. Some kids just want to do things when they feel like it.

I have seen all kinds of children over my 40 plus years of training and teaching martial arts.

4

THE AGGRESSIVE CHILD

For kids who are aggressive, they are taught to only hit the pads not another person. Hitting the pads channels their aggression in a positive way. A focus pad can be hit as hard as a student can hit and no one gets hurt. Maybe the kid stubs his toe if he hits the pad the wrong way, but they soon learn to focus and hit it correctly and pay attention to the instructor who is telling them how to do it right.

I have found that most of the time the "aggressive child" simply has a *following direction* problem. They want to do it right away right now and only pick up on certain words of whatever command or instruction is given. For example, if I tell the student to do a kicking combination, let's say "front kick right leg, front kick left leg, and punch then go to the end of the line" he might only hear "kick and punch" and wants to keep going instead of taking only his turn. He never heard "go to the end of the line" part of the command. It is the same when a parent says "Johnny clean up your toys right now so we can get going to Grandma's house." Johnny only hears "Johnny, toys to Grandma's house." And parents wonder "why is he taking his dinosaur with him while leaving the room a mess, doesn't he know we are in a hurry?"

If Johnny is 3 or 4 years old he might not have the capability to mentally understand all the word and the context which was intended.

5

THE SHY CHILD

Confidence comes over time with martial arts training. Remember we are talking about being shy not withdrawn. If the child is withdrawn then I recommend a licensed therapist or psychiatrist. Martial arts doesn't fix everything and everyone. Right now, we are talking about a child who is shy meaning a little reluctant to try new things and or socialize with others.

This one is not as hard as it sounds. All the child has to do is try and have fun in the process and then he or she comes out of his or her shell. Once he or she sees how easy and fun martial arts is, then they slowly start to socialize with other kids and make friends. I've seen it hundreds of times.

Think about it. Not everyone does martial arts. It is unique to say the least. If it were "main stream" then everyone would know how to do it. A martial art class would be part of elementary school recess like kickball or dodge ball. In Korea, they do Tae Kwon Do as part of their education system.

So, a shy child feels different and unique practicing martial arts. They learn cool kicks, punches, forms (patterns designed to help with memorization, power, speed, timing etc.) and get to break boards. And no, they do not get hurt breaking boards. Here at Karate Universe we use boards proportionate to the student's size. Obviously a 3 or 4-year-old wouldn't break a board proportionate to an adult or a teenager and vice versa. Let's face it, an adult breaking a tiny board would look a little ridiculous.

With the proper training and motivation, the shy child goes from hesitating to realizing they do things (breaking, forms, jump kicks, spin kicks etc.) that other people cannot do and then they feel a sense of accomplishment which in turns gives them confidence.

I have taught hundreds if not thousands of shy children. Three children spring to mind. One boy Connor was extremely shy. He had a curious mind as most 4-year olds do, and always wanted to know things about me, martial arts, when he can use weapons, etc. However, the thing was he wouldn't ask directly. Instead, he would whisper what he wanted to know, to his mother, who he'd be sitting next to in our waiting area. He would purposely make his mother show up early before class would start just to ask stuff he wanted to know of course whispering it all to his mom. His mom would always be like "you ask him". This went on for a few years and then one day he popped out of his shy shell and started talking to everyone, me, other students, other instructors, everyone and anyone. You couldn't get him to stop talking. He became very outgoing, very confident and made it to 3rd degree black belt here at Karate Universe before he went to college. Needless to say, he is a student I am very fond and proud of.

The other two children were twin girls. Their names are Kiara and Katrina. Both girls were extremely shy. They started when they were four years old. You want to talk about shy girls? They wouldn't even look at me when I was teaching them. They would just smile and sometimes look at each other and giggle. I don't remember exactly when they came out of their shells but both came out at the same time. After training only one year here at Karate Universe, they did a complete 180-degree transformation. They were talking, looking at you when you spoke to them; they had the confidence every parent dreams of for their children. They were so confident they would plot to "attack" me. One twin would be jumping off equipment and latching onto my back while the other one tackled my legs trying to knock me down. They felt extremely comfortable with me as their instructor and so confident they would yell "jump on sir day" to rally all the other kids in class to help them. Please realize this was before class even started. Once I started class all their shenanigans stopped and they were model students for the entire class. Obviously, our program works on shy children, and as these girls grew up they became leaders among their peers, were able to excel in martial arts with great ability to defend themselves to the point where none of the male students wanted to spar them or be their self defense partner. Katrina earned her third-degree black belt and Kiara earned her second-degree black belt. Kiara wanted to focus on her studies to get into Harvard instead of obtaining her third-degree black belt. Talk about goal setting (we will talk about goal setting later in this book) and focusing. And they were able to focus so well they did fantastic academically and Kiara did go to Harvard. In fact, they both are now Medical Doctors. They are two of Karate Universe's finest students becoming very successful in life. Everyone at Karate Universe is proud of them and their accomplishments and I thank their parents for letting me watch them grow up from age 4 all the way to they went off to college. Needless to say, they are apart of our Karate Universe family forever.

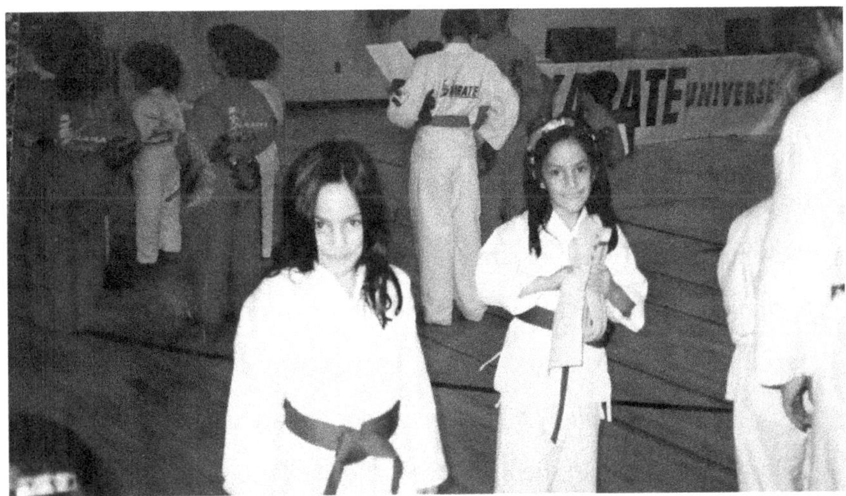

6

THE KID WHO DOES WHAT HE WANTS

This is the kid who just doesn't listen or respect what mom or dad say. Threats don't faze him/her and they feel they can do what they want when they want. All children will push parents to see what their limits are. This happens with all ages from 3-year old all the way to teenagers. Pushing to find their limit is natural and part of child development. Martial art training teaches respect, listening to parents, and being able to follow directions. Here at Karate Universe when a child doesn't listen to the instructors they have to deal with the consequences (time outs, not being able to promote, reduced in rank), just like when they do listen they get rewarded (getting to participate in the "game/drill", able to promote, getting to participate in special events, etc). Kids crave structure and discipline. They want to know what their boundaries are and what is right and wrong. This has to be reinforced at home. This doesn't mean a parent doesn't love their child if they discipline them, just the opposite it means you love them enough to guide them in the right direction in life. Jails are full of people who cannot follow rules and laws. Parents need to parent and not try to be their child's friend. Instructors are fair but firm which is why they listen to and respect the instructors. Instructors are consistent with both the way they treat each student as well as if the student behaves proper or not. It is this consistency children want and crave. Parents must have the same consistency with their rules and consequences. Something can't be okay one day and not okay a month later. Or okay one time and then no longer allowed. That sends mixed messages to the child, confusing them in the process. The confusion will then cause the child to act out because they can't understand the change. Depending on age they may lack the capacity to understand the change being too young.

I have had parents tell me that they just can't "punish" their child because they feel too guilty for not spending enough time with them. I know life is hectic for parents trying to balance their own life with career and family, but being consistent with your child's behavior is paramount. My grandfather always said the days are long but the years are short. You only get so many impressionable years with your child; shouldn't you make them count by being consistent? If you do then your child will respect you, admire you and when they become an adult or a parent, they will thank you for all you did showing them right from wrong.

There is also the flip side of parents being over protective for their child and do everything for them. If parents do everything for their child, the child never learns responsibility, never gets to make mistakes and learn from their mistakes. Children won't listen or respect their parent when the parent tells them to do something because the child knows mom or dad will eventually do it because they do everything for them. Parents cannot shelter their children from getting bumps and bruises in life. As an instructor, I allow my students to make mistakes on their techniques and correct their mistake. If a student falls down doing a kick, I tell them to get up and keep their hands up for balance and do it again. Instructors don't coddle students because we know students will get black and blues, cuts or scrapes (in our case mat burns) both literally and figuratively because life is hard. Children need to learn that as they develop so they can handle what the world dishes out to them as adults.

Parents should *work with* the instructor to help make their child better. If there is an issue or a problem then the parent should work *with* the instructor to fix it. An instructor has the experience of years if not decades teaching children. Too many times a parent will come to me and say "We are pulling Johnny out of Karate since he's not listening to us at home". At that point, it is too late for an instructor to help correct Johnny's behavior. It is also the wrong thing to do because martial arts get children to become better listeners. If a parent has an issue with Johnny let the instructor know IMMEDIATELY! Together we can find the cause and fix the issue before it becomes a major problem out of control. Children do not come with instructions like kitchen appliances. The old saying two heads are better than one does work. Many times, over the years, I have given strategies or solutions to help the parent. Sometimes I have had to talk to the student with the parent explaining why xyz behavior is unacceptable. Sometimes having another person, the child looks up to as a role model helps drive the point home for the child to understand what the correct thing to do is. So why not use the martial art instructor as a <u>resource to help?</u> I am not saying the instructor take over as a substitute parent (not always being "the heavy", and the parent saying "I'll tell your instructor you are not listening to me" etc.) All I am suggesting is to use our **influence** to your benefit with your child's behavior. After all we are one of your child's role models in their life, just like their teachers in school, you their parents, their grandparents etc. Some kids act like we are super-heroes and think martial arts is like having super powers because we break boards, do spinning and jump kicks so high...only if we really could fly.

So that is why here at Karate Universe we start them so young. Like stated before, little kids little problems, big kids big problems. Children become physically fit, mentally strong, know how to pick and keep good friends and learn to do the right things in life here at Karate Universe.

7

SIDE BAR – WHERE ARE MANNERS TAUGHT?

We also make sure all students use their proper manners at a young age. Personally, I don't help any student with equipment, uniform, belt or anything else unless they say "Please Sir". A 4-year-old white belt will come up to me with his belt that fell off him in his hand and show me the belt fell off. When I ask him "what do you need?" the usual answer is "my belt". I then agree that the belt is his and then he usually says "it fell off". Then I respond with "and?" and the kid says "tie it". I will then say "how do you ask?" and they respond "tie my belt" which I then say "no". The looks I have gotten over the years are priceless; confused, puzzled, shock, and even the "how dare you" look from a 4-year-old. (Children should realize adults should be respected and adults are not the child's servants and taken for granted). I then of course coach them on the proper way of asking; asking them if they know the "magic words" which then either clicks with the child who then uses the word "Please". Some children I have encountered over the years were never taught by anyone to say please. I sometimes wonder if common courtesy is no longer taught to these children. Years ago, one mom would consistently stay on top of her children to say please, thank you; excuse me, and Yes Mr. Jones, No Mrs. Smith. What struck me was the way she did it always asking "what do you say?" Her children were the most well-mannered children I have ever had the privilege of teaching. Brandon and Lauren were so well mannered they always did the right thing. They never had any behavior issues. They were just on the shy side and did come out of their shells as well like the examples above. Thank you, Mrs. Barbara D, for teaching me how to ask children about pleases and thank you, you were my role model in this area of life. Even a master instructor can learn from a student.

Again, insisting a child says please is discipline, not being mean or cruel. Having the child say "please and thank you" should be done by age 2, in my opinion by the parents. Please keep in mind just like a doctor works hard to earn their PHD and is referred to as "Doctor", an instructor works hard to earn their level of black belt and should be referred to as "Sir". Both titles deserve respect for their respective accomplishments. This is just common courtesy and civility being taught, not ego or cruelty. Respect is the Martial Art way.

8

SO, KARATE IS THE BEST STYLE TO SIGN UP MY KID?

There is no best style. Here at Karate Universe our main discipline is Tae Kwon Do. To be more specific we belong to the World Tae Kwon Do Federation. The World Tae Kwon Do Federation (WTF for short), is the only martial art taught in over 200 countries around the world. The WTF is recognized by the United States Olympic Committee (USOC) and the International Olympic Committee (IOC) and is an Olympic event during the summer games. We have had students move to India, Brussels, Florida, California, Minnesota, etc and not have to start over again. (See Appendix for History of Tae Kwon Do)

We also do the best of all the other styles (Karate, Kung Fu, Arnis, Hapkido etc.) as well as all the Chinese, Japanese and Philippine weaponry. Weapons are the ultimate test of self control and self discipline. You have to know your distance from other people and objects. You have to be aware of your surroundings and be able to control the weapon. You are in control of the weapon, the weapon is not in control of you. After all, martial art weapons are an extension of the student's hand. Of course, beginners do not do weaponry. That would be stupid. Students first need to learn the basics of martial arts and be able to control their kicks and punches. They need to control themselves first before even attempting weapons. As an instructor, it is one of my responsibilities to make sure the student is never put in harm's way and yet at the same time keep challenging the student for their skill to progress. Talk about balancing because every student is unique and different; never mind the fact that there are different ages and belt ranks.

9
BELT RANKS

Often a new parent will ask what the entire belt system means. There are many explanations I have heard over the decades…white belt symbolizes purity or a blank foundation, Blue represents the sky etc. Frankly speaking martial art suppliers have created different colors, striping, multi-colored belts because they now have the technology and know how. Now all colors on the spectrum are offered to martial art academies; including Pink. It's at this time I want to point out and apologize to Melissa, Kristen and all the other little girls who asked me for a pink belt in the 1990's. They just didn't have it back then, sorry.

To be direct the belt system is really for the instructors to know what curriculum is introduced at what time of the student's life. Basically, it is so we know what to teach each student. Obviously, a beginner shouldn't do certain techniques due to lack of experience and the complexity of certain techniques and the fact that they are not in the physical condition required to accomplish the technique efficiently or accurately. A person would expect a high-ranking belt say a red or brown belt to be able to perform difficult jump kicks, flying side kicks, etc. again due to the fact of their physical conditioning, experience and duration of practicing their martial art.

For students, each rank is a goal to accomplish. They set a goal: their next belt rank, work on the required material, practice and perfect said material and then are tested on their skill level and understanding of the requirements. This is goal setting at its finest. Set a goal and work to achieve it period. And of course, parents want this to expand in all aspects of their child's life, school, sports, etc. which it does because it becomes a process and a habit for the student.

Now many parents always want to know when my kid is ready to test. Here at Karate Universe we only test 3 times per year and we only send children to test when the instructors say they are ready to promote. An old saying is "when the student is ready the master will appear". Well we modified it to "when the student is ready the testing papers will appear" meaning the instructors will give the test papers.

Obviously, the student must meet all requirements set before them. Each martial art style and academy is different. Some require physical ability e.g. certain number or push ups, being able to run an 8-minute mile, being able to jump over a person and perform a tuck and roll. Other styles and academies want memorization of every form, self defense, the student was ever taught. And others just want you to show up and you pass. The level of commitment and expectations on both the parents and the child should be in agreement with the instructor ahead of time.

Karate Universe requires each student to do their best, be proficient in all testing requirements: Forms, Self-defense (depending on age), and Sparring (for low belts no contact), and Breaking (an age appropriate board).

In my opinion, all students should be able to kick at least their own head level which requires a student to have a fantastic stretch. If children/students can do a split, then more power to them because when they are adults, their legs will be in excellent condition to be able to defend themselves despite the natural aging process which takes away a person's flexibility. By doing all the stretching when a student is young provides longevity when the student reaches an age past their prime.

My instructors taught me that Tae Kwon Do is a loving art and a giving art. I know this is true because I have seen it happen to one of my students: Penelope.

This was a little girl whose parents brought her to Karate Universe when she was four years old. Yes, she was a little shy, but Penelope had a physical issue, she would fall every three to four feet when she walked. One summer day, Penelope was in shorts and her mom asked if she could use our restroom to get her changed into her uniform for class. Of course, I let her do so but I couldn't believe how many bruises were on her legs. There was no exaggeration about this child falling down every few feet. In fact, Yale Hospital located in New Haven Connecticut was ready to put this child in leg braces for the rest of her life. It reminded me of the movie Forrest Gump, but this was real life and this was a student right in front of me. It was because of our program and training and stretching, that her legs got stronger, her bone density increased and she did NOT have to have her legs in braces.

She was even able to do the spinning kicks and jumping kicks like all the other students. We never treated her any different than the other kids and she excelled becoming a Second Degree Black Belt before going off to college. She was a very dedicated and wonderful student who to this very day I am extremely proud of her.

The styles and instructors who put physical requirements like running, pushups, jumping over a person etc. allow only the physically strong young 18 to 25-year old able to become a black belt. That is the same age for military service as well as most people's prime in their lives. Tae Kwon Do can be done by everyone all ages no matter what shape or size you are. Students get better in time. Better physical condition, better mental health, better emotional development as well as social development through our Tae Kwon Do program here at Karate Universe.

SO, MARTIAL ARTS IS JUST FOR KIDS
THE STORY OF RON

Now at this point of this book, you are probably thinking that martial arts are only for children. Although, the vast majority of students are children, adults can and do practice martial arts as well, with tremendous success.

This brings me to one of my adult students named Ron. Ron was a typical person, husband, married with three children, had a typical job, out of shape, over-weight, a cigarette smoker, not very motivated in general. Ron knew he should take better care of himself. Ron was over six feet tall and easily weighed over 250 pounds. He tried every program, gym, fad that was out there. He came to Karate Universe looking for a change, and change is exactly what he got. He would literally drag himself to class. I would see him enter our doors looking tired and weary. He would literally flop into a chair in our waiting area and take ten-minutes to take off his shoes before heading to the changing area. I felt bad for him but I didn't take it easy on him during class. I would motivate him to do better, kick stronger, give it his all, and complimented him on achieving the task at hand. After classes, he would always tell me how he felt so much better, had a little more energy than when he first walked in to Karate Universe. After a few years, I got him to stop smoking simply by pointing out how much better he would be if he stopped and his stamina would increase exponentially. Ron was worried once he quit smoking he would then gain some more weight. Well I am happy to say he actually lost 40 pounds after he stopped smoking and was under 200 pounds by the time he was ready to test for his Black Belt. Ron would always thank me after classes for my patience, understanding, and motivation. I was a young instructor at the time and was just happy to help him out. He did a complete transformation compared to when he first started with us. Physically, he lost weight and got into better health and a healthy life-style. Mentally, he was able to focus on work better getting promoted at his job. His family life improved dramatically, he became a better husband and father to his wife and kids.

Ron found balance in his life and things seemed to be going his way. Then one day, he walked in to Karate Universe in a somber state. He took class as usual, did great as usual and then after class he hung back asking if I had a few minutes to talk. I asked what was on his mind and then he told me. Apparently, he was doing so well at work he was getting noticed among his companies' competitors as well as all his peers in his industry. Ron told me he was approached by some investors. These investors wanted Ron to be the CEO (Chief Executive Officer) of their new company they had just started. Ron then told me their offer, they offered to buy his existing house, help him relocate him to Pennsylvania, pay for all his moving expenses, give him a company car, they found the best private schools for all three of his children and as Ron put it "they offered him an obscene amount of money." I then asked Ron what was the problem and he said, he did not know what to do. First, I asked him if he could handle the job they offered him as CEO. He confidently without any hesitation said he could absolutely do the job. Second, I asked Ron, would this be a better life for his family. Again, confidently and without any hesitation said absolutely. So, I then asked him what was the problem and like a light switch turning on I saw his eyes light up. His statement to me was "Wow, you make it so simple." Needless to say, he did take the job and relocated his family to Pennsylvania. Below is a thank you letter from Ron.

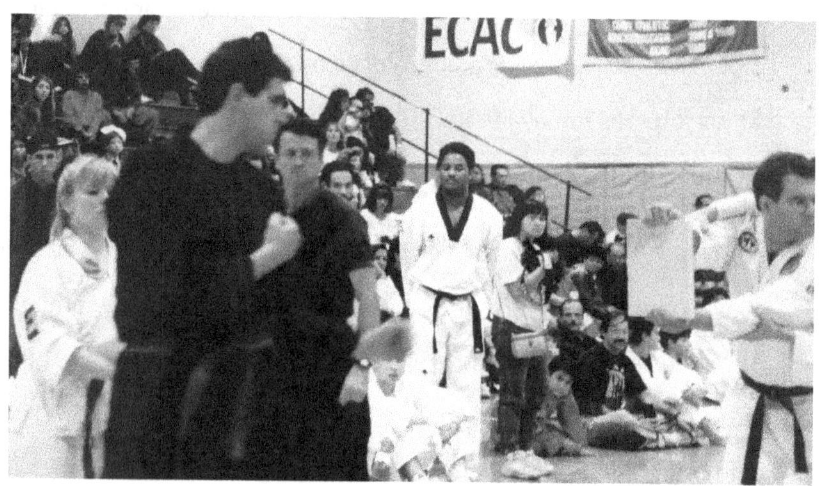

Dear Master Spiros and Master Dean,

As my association with Karate Universe begins to moderate because of a job change requiring relocation, I felt compelled to write to you and express my deepest thanks for all that you communication medium for what I have to express but I shall try anyway.

Tomorrow my rank will change from Bo-Dan to 1st Degree Black Belt. This change will occur for two (2) primary reasons: 1. You, and 2. Me.

Yes, I have worked very hard for this ultimate honor for I did not bring much physical talent to the process but, you are far more responsible than me for my accomplishments. Your contributions to me went well beyond the excellent physical training program of the academy. What I will always remember and cherish is your absolute refusal to give up on me as a student during times of physical or metal lapses over the past 4 years. There were times when I might have given up on myself but you simply refused to let that happen. This, more than anything else, gives richness to my memories and experience of Karate Universe.

I know who I am. I know what I want to be. I know how to get there. This knowingness of self, this clarity of thought and this single mindedness of purpose is directly attributable to your teachings and your sharing and caring spirit.

I plan to continue my training in Pennsylvania but I will never forget and will always cherish Karate Universe. I will not suggest that my skills include clairvoyance but, somehow in my heart I know that the moderation of my association with you is temporary. I will return to my beloved academy.

Master Spiros, I love you as I would love a father and respect you as a Master.

Master Dean, I love you as I would love a brother and respect you as a Master. Thank you for the patience, the training and the experience.

You Forever Respectful, Thankful and Loyal Student

Ron

11

RESPECT HAS TO BE INSTILLED AT A YOUNG AGE

So far, in this book we have covered young children starting martial arts. We have stated that doing the right thing from a young age becomes a habit. We've said children need to learn to respect their parents, teachers, elders, brothers and sisters, friends and most importantly themselves. If they cannot respect themselves it is almost impossible for them to respect any one else.

As children grow and develop and get older, they are influenced by sources outside the family unit. Social media is huge among pre-teen and teenagers. Pop culture decides what is "cool" or "in style" and no longer is the parent's opinion valued as much. The older kids at school influence your child. Television and movie celebrities and professional athletes are looked up to; but are they the best role models for your children? How many of these "celebrities" have a drug or alcohol addiction? Parents cannot protect their children from harmful influences twenty-four hours a day. You as a parent, try to instill good values in your child. You want them to do the right things in life. You want them to stay away from drugs and alcohol. Parents know the destructiveness drugs and alcohol can cause a person and you don't want it to be your child. You want them to make good choices as they grow up.

I can safely say yes, they can make the right choices in life. I was not born a master instructor. I grew up in NYC. I did martial arts since I was four-years old. I had school friends, neighborhood friends, and my martial art friends growing up. I can tell you from my personal experience that doing the right thing from a young age does indeed become a habit. My instructors got me to believe in myself. That I can achieve and do things that I thought I never could do. I was taught how to concentrate and focus. One of the most important lessons I was taught was to realize I didn't have to prove anything to anybody. It was that lesson which kept me out of trouble growing up, staying away from drugs and alcohol. I didn't care what my school friends did; if they went to a party to drink beers or do drugs, or steal something on a dare. My martial art friends had the same value system that I did and we hung out together going to the movies, pizza, training together, etc. We helped keep each other in check so we didn't disappoint our parents and our instructors as well.

It is these lessons that I now teach my student and the same habit of doing the right things in life has helped them become successful in life. I get my student to believe in themselves. That they can achieve and do things that they thought they could not do. I teach them to focus and concentrate and constantly tell them they do not have to prove anything to anybody. I also, teach them to realize they can always do better and that they should not rest on their accomplishments. After all the biggest room in the world is the room of improvement!

My students learn they need to condition their body and stay healthy for the long term; for their longevity. They learn to look at things logically and examine their skills to stay sharp. I teach my black belts how to protect themselves by showing them where to hit and how to strike an opponent. I also remind my black belts to not start a fight but if it is necessary to fight then make sure they win a fight. I tell all my black belts to ask themselves questions when they wish to improve their techniques. Am I kicking high enough? , Is my stance correct or am I off balance? And most importantly, they should find balance in their lives. Not just balance in martial arts, but balance between, school, friends, sports, family, martial art training, and anything else they do in life. They learn if they put their mind to something then it WILL happen. Whether it be achieving a goal such as black belt, or getting a hundred on a spelling test they can make it happen. If the student wants to get a split or do 100 pushups in 60 seconds, then it is their mind telling the body what to do. If they really want it and believe that they can do it then it does happen. They also learn to respect themselves, their parents, elders, teachers, brothers and sister (yes they have to get along with their siblings) and are reminded of these lessons every class they train here at Karate Universe.

12
LEVEL OF COMMITMENT

Now you are probably asking yourself what type of commitment is all this? Well, what level of commitment do you make in raising your child? Remember you want your child to be a better version of themselves. There is no instant potion to make this transformation and there is always room for improving one-self. Rome was not built in one day and it took thousands of years to become a beautiful city. It does take years to be proficient at anything. If I can jump in a time machine with you and show you what your child will be like in say, four years, you would be amazed. Your child's physical skills, agility, speed, strength, weight control, flexibility, coordination; their mental skills, focus, concentration, alertness, listening skills; their social and emotional skills, confidence, self-discipline, positive attitude, self-esteem, assertiveness, pride, integrity would totally and utterly exceed all of your expectations.

Where a student starts as a white belt is totally different (physically, mentally, socially, and emotionally) by the time they become a black belt. This transformation may not look drastic over time but if you were able to put the white belt student standing next to the same student as a black belt you would literally see night and day differences of the same individual.

As a parent, you will experience both joys and challenges during your child's journey to Black Belt. Remember, ALL children like to push their boundaries. There will be times your child will say he or she doesn't want to do martial arts. Just like I am sure they tell you they don't want to go to school or they don't want to brush their teeth. Yet parents always make their children go to school and brush their teeth because they know it is good for them. If you gave a sick child a choice of medicine or candy to feel better they most likely will choose the candy even though the medicine which has value will make them well. Everyone has ups and downs like a rollercoaster. You feel great one day, lousy the next and then super the following day. This is part of human nature. You can't let your children quit in life. If they give up in martial arts, then they give up in sports, school (imagine paying three and a half years of college and your child tells you he or she is quitting college; you would want to kill them), relationships, marriages, abandon their children (your grandchildren) because everything is too hard. It becomes a domino affect, they look for an out, withdrawal from their normal life and seek something which will make them feel good even if it is temporary – they turn to drugs. This isn't as extreme as it sounds because I have witnessed former students who stopped training with us in the local paper's police blotter. These were the parents who said they didn't want to "force" their child to do it or they pulled out of the program because they weren't listening to the parent and that was a form of punishment – not going to martial art classes.

Parents, you have to be committed before your child can commit. They can't drive. Sometimes a parent feels that their job is to be a taxi cab drive and sometimes the taxi driver doesn't want to go unless the kid begs. A parent's job is to set the child's life rules and to nurture the child until the rules are part of the child's value system. Parents, let us face a cold, hard fact. You are ultimately responsible for designing, developing and instilling your child's value system. Train a child in the way he should go and when he is older, he will not deviate from it. Look at any news broadcast. When a child turns out to be worthless, the parents are blamed, but when your child turns out to be priceless, you will be praised.

Remember to work with your child's martial art instructor. Instructors are a parental resource. Instructors are very committed to making their students better. We want our students to succeed. We want your children to succeed. We understand that some techniques, forms, board break, etc. are difficult. How to we know, because we have been there. We persevered and know the student can persevere also. We don't give up on you and your child, so don't give up on us. We understand how your child feels if they have been on vacation and are worried they missed things they don't know what or how to do them. We have patience and understanding. We can break down the difficult so your child won't feel overwhelmed. We feel for our students. We are troubled when they fail and we rejoice on their successes. Let's make them successful in life!

May you and your child's vision of me tying their Black Belt around him soon become a reality!

Yours in Martial Arts

Master Dean

APPENDIX

A General Introduction

Tae Kwon Do literally means "the way of kicking and punching" (Tae = 'To kick', Kwon = 'to punch' and Do = 'art, or the way'). Its techniques were devleoped and perfected over many centuries out of the basic need for protection against enemy attacks. Humankind's most basic instinct is that of survival, and at a time when no other means of defense existed, bare hands skills were the difference between life and death. As human-kind developed tools, weapons were also developed (many based on farm tools), but even then people devoted themselves to developing physical strength and skills. Tae Kwon Do developed from this basic need of survival into a complete system of self-defense and personal improvement whose sharp strong angular movements combined with smooth circular movements produce a balance of beauty and power.

Is TaeKwonDo dangerous?

TaeKwonDo is a full-contact sport and much care must be taken to avoid injury. Proper techniques and training ensure control and help prevent injuries. At Karate Universe it is your option to participate in full contact sparring or non-contact sparring.

Karate Universe also teaches "traditional" Tae Kwon Do!

History of TaeKwonDo

The earliest records of Martial Arts practice in Korea date back to 50 B.C. This ancient form of Martial Art was known as 'Tae Kyon'. Evidence of 'Tae Kyon' can be found in tombs and temples where wall-paintings and carvings show men in fighting-stances. One such example can be found on a tower wall of a Buddhist temple over two thousand years old in what is now Korea. Two giant figures were carved facing each other in fighting stances as if in the middle of a Martial Art's fight. Another example can be found in a painting on the ceiling of the Muyong-Chong, a royal tomb from the Koguryu dynasty. Such evidence typically show unarmed man in combat stances using techniques that closely resemble those of modern Tae Kwon Do. The knife hand, closed fist and some classical stances predominate in paintings and carvings of that era.

During that period there co-existed 3 kingdoms in what is now Korea:

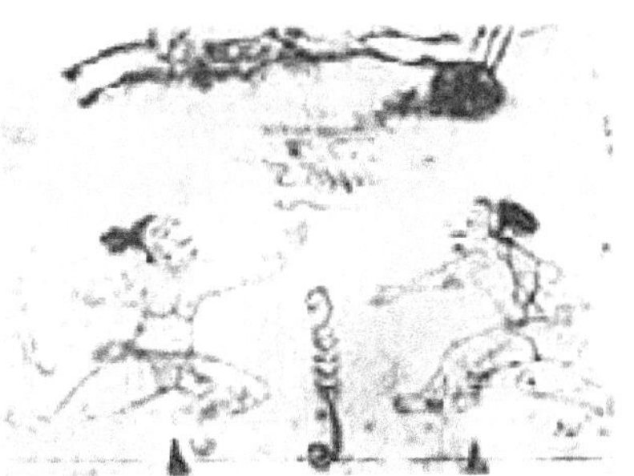

1. Koguryo (37 B.C. - A.D. 668)
2. Paekje (18 B.C. - A.D. 600)
3. Shilla (57 B.C. - A.D. 935)

Out of three kingdoms, Shilla was the first to be formed, but remained the smallest and less civilized.

Shilla was constantly under attack by Japanese pirates, and armed forces were sent from Koguryu to lend a hand in the fights against the pirates. It was then that Taek Kyon was introduced to the Shilla's armed forces by early masters known as the Sonbae.

The Shilla warriors trained in Taek Kyon became known as Hwarang. The Hwarang established a military academy for the young nobility, and later became a society known as Hwarang-Do, which means "the way of the flowering youth" (Hwa="flower", Rang="Young Man", Do="the way"). This society comprised of an elite group of young men, devoted to cultivating mind and body and serve the kingdom.

The Hwarang practiced various forms of martial arts, which included Taek Kyon as part of the basic training, and had an honor-code that became the philosophical background to Tae Kwon Do. Besides martial arts the Hwanrang were trained in many more disciplines. Disciplines such as history, Confucian philosophy, ethics, Buddhist morality, horse riding, archery, and military tactics were all part of the rigorous Hwanrang-Do training. This rigorous training and the Hwanrang-Do honor code were based on the Five Codes of Human Conduct, as established by Buddhist scholars:

* Be loyal to your country
* Be obedient to your parents
* Be trustworthy to your friends
* Never retreat in battle
* Never make an unjust kill

During the time of peace following the unification of the three kingdoms, the Hwarang turned from military training to poetry and music. During this time the Hwarang traveled throughout the peninsula in order to learn more about the kingdom and its people. The Taek Kyon's focus was turned from a military discipline into a sport and recreational activity designed to improve physical fitness as the Hwarang spread it across the region. In 936 A.D. the Koryo dynasty (abbreviation of Koguryo) was founded and Taek Kyon focus was reshifted (the name Korea is derived from the word Koryo). The Taek Kyon evolved into Subakhu (Taek Kyon contests) and it's popularity among the masses increased. It became a more systemized Martial Art, divided into basic moves and hand and foot techniques. The importance of Taek Kyon during the Koryo grew greatly. During this dynasty it became common for plain soldiers who mastered Taek Kyon to become generals. At the same time young Taek Kyon practitioners became military officers by demonstrating their skills through Taek Kyon contests.

With the advent of the Yi Dynasty (1392 A.D - 1910 A.D.) the emphasis on military training for the young nobility disappeared and the art became popular among the general population thanks to the first widely available book on Martial Arts. The development of

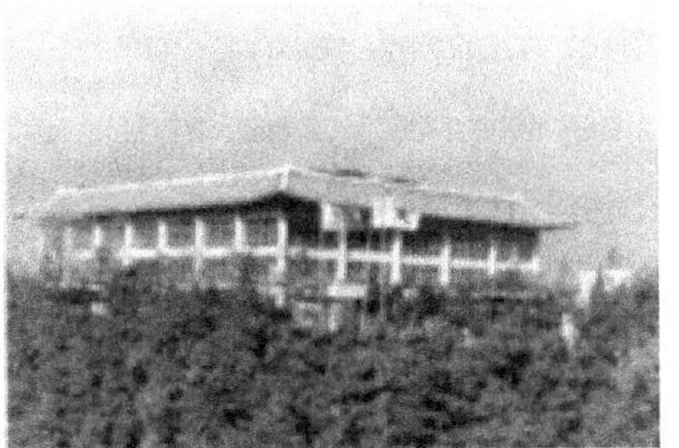

gunpowder and new types of
weapons caused a loss of
popularity of the Subakhu Do.

Taek Kyon and Subakhu survived only in a few families which handed down the art from generation to generation until the end of the 16th century when the need of a strong defense system was revived. From 1910 to the end of World War II Korea was ruled by Japan which fearful of population uprisings, and eager to wipe out all traces of Korean culture, banned the practice of Korean martial arts.

This ban only increased interest and renewed the growth of the Subakhu Do, and it survived through secretly being taught in secret schools. This continued until 1943 when other martial arts were introduced in the country, bringing Subakhu out of the shadows back into the lives of the Korean people. The introduction of Japanese Karate in Korea eventually influenced the Subakhu Do, which assimilated some of the quick straight-line movements that characterize Japanese martial art systems. Some of this assimilation was no doubt fueled by the training that many Korean soldiers received in Japan. After the liberation of Korea, at the end of W.W. II several schools teaching native Korean Martial Arts were opened during the period prior to the early 1960's.

Differences in the teachings among the many schools (Kwan) prevented the formation of regulatory boards, but after a half-hour demonstration in 1952 the president of Korea ordered training in the Martial Arts to be adopted as part of basic military training. Fueled by the acceptance of the traditional Korean Martial Arts by the military a meeting was convened in 1955 to attempt the unification of the many Kwans under a common name. Tae Soo Do was initially accepted, but two years later the name was changed to Tae Kwon Do. There were two main reasons for the adoption of the name Tae Kwon Do: it accurately describes the nature of the art and it resembles the art's early name, Taek Kyon.

In 1961 the Korean TaeKwonDo Union was formed, and in 1962 it was acknowledged and became a member of the Korean Amateur Sports Association. In 1964 the name was set to Korean TaeKwonDo Association (K.T.A.) and an international association was formed. Demonstrations were given all over the world, but little progress was made,
but in 1973 the World TaeKwonDo Federation was founded and the first biennial International WTF championships were held in Soul. Since then World Championships have been held all over the world. In 1980 Tae Kwon Do was introduced to the International Olympic Committee and Tae Kwon Do as a sport became an official Demonstration Sport for the 1988 Olympics Games in Seoul, Korea. Tae Kwon Do has since become an official Olympic sport starting in the Olympic Games of 2000 in Sydney, Australia. Tae Kwon Do is officially practiced by over 20 million people in 166 countries.

I.T.F vs W.T.F
After a goodwill trip to North-Korea in 1966 General Choi, one of the original officials of the KTA, fell in disgrace in the eyes of

the South-Koreans and resigned his post in the KTA. ITF TaeKwonDo concentrates on forms developed by General Choi himself.

Its focus is on forms and semi-contact sparring.

Meantime the KTA expanded itself internationally in 1973 with the formation of the WTF(World TaeKwonDo Federation). The WTF initially concentrated on the Palgwe forms, and later changed from the Palgwes and started concentrating on the TaeGuks. Recognition to the WTF came when TaeKwonDo was admitted as a sport in the 2000 Olympiads in Sydney, Australia. Only members of the WTF organization are allowed to compete in the TaeKwonDo competition in the Olympic Games.

Since the original break-up (General Choi and KTA) attempts to reunite the two most recognized TaeKwonDo Federations, have had no sucess. WTF and ITF insiders and practitioners alike fear that a Union between these two federations may not be possible. Especially since only the World TaeKwonDo Federation is sanctioned by the International Olympic Committee, Karate Universe is an International Olympic

Commitee sanctioned Martial Arts School via, its association with the WTF family.

Ethics and TaeKwonDo

Ethics are a component of the utmost importance in all Martial Arts, and that is especially true for TaeKwonDo. Respect, Loyalty and Morality are of the most importance to TaeKwonDo and are expressed daily in the life of the TaeKwonDo student.

Training of TaeKwonDo shapes not only the physical aspects of the body, but more importantly it goes deep into the soul. Balance and harmony with oneself as well as nature are the most basic principles in the TaeKwonDo knowledge book. This balance is gained with the control of both good and evil (the concept of Ying Vs. Yang found in so many philosophy and religious teachings from the Far East). The ability to recognize both Ying and Yang forces gives the TaeKwonDo student the ability to know how to behave in all situations. The idea that TaeKwonDo is merely a collection of self-defense techniques, or a means to achieve superiority over others could not be any further from the Truth. TaeKwonDo is a way of life. The respect relationship between master and student goes beyond the confines of the Dojang (TaeKwonDo gym) and expresses itself in respect towards others. Humility is another quality the serious student will possess. Although TaeKwonDo boosts self-confidence it should not reflect itself in a sense of superiority towards others. The true student will avoid confrontation at all costs and only make use of its skills on others in self-defense.

TaeKwonDo Etiquette's

TaeKwonDo has a general set of rules, or codes, which all students must follow. These codes are strongly influenced by Buddishm and are reflected in the modern 'Commandments of TaeKwonDo'. The influence on the modern commandments comes from the Hwarans Do code of honor:

The modern commandments of TaeKwonDo are used as a guide for moral development. No student that does not fully understand and live these tenets can ever hope to master the true essence of TaeKwonDo. The twelve commandments of TaeKwonDo are:

1. Loyalty to your country
2. Respect your parents
3. Faithfulness to your spouse
4. Respect you brothers and sisters
5. Loyalty to your friends
6. Respect your elders
7. Respect your teachers
8. Never take life unjustly
9. Indomitable spirit
10. Loyalty to your school
11. Finish what you begin
12. Say no to drugs and no to smoking

We teach beyond punching and kicking. We maximize human potential!

- **Karate Universe**

ABOUT THE AUTHOR

<u>Credentials:</u>

7th Dan World Tae Kwon Do Kukkiwon Certified No_09902063

XMA Licensed Instructor ; (Extreme Martial Arts)

Studied at Shaolin Temple in Togo, China; learned Chinese Boxing Form & Mantis

Versed in both Pyn ahn, Palgwe and Taeguek Forms

Martial Art Weapons Expert:

   Single Nunchuk, Double Nunchuk, Single Broad Sword, Double Broad Sword, Bo Staff, Kamas, Sais, Kwan Dao, Twin Tiger Hook Swords, Butterfly Swords, Arnis, Tonfa, Cane

Experience with 3 Section Staff, Katana Sword, Chinese Whip

Mu Tai, Hapkido and Grapple experience

<u>Accomplishments in Martial Arts</u>

12/20/92 Referee Certification D-3

03/04/94 Referee Certificate of Participation of referee seminar hosted in Rhode Island by Grand Master Jin Hong

03/09/96 Rhode Island State Championship Silver Medal Poomse

05/09/96 Participated in 22nd National Taekwondo Championship

10/12/96 US Cup Taekwondo Championship Silver Medal Poomse

05/04/02 Certificate of License

Master Instructor License

10/06/02 Coach at 2002 USTU President's Cup in New Jersey

10/25/09 Participated and assisted in PATU Poomse Seminar conducted by Grand Master Ji Ho Choi

11/08/09 WTF Citation for promoting Taekwondo

11/21/10 Referee at Eastern Collegiate Taekwondo Tournament held in Princeton NJ

2003 – Current Coach at Big East Tournament

2003 – Current Coach at Garden State Championship Tournament

09/27/14 Participated in Kukkiwon Poomse Seminar hosted at White Tiger in Cary, NC

2004 – 2016 Best Instructor Award Big East Tournament

2004 – 2016 Best Instructor Award Garden State Championship Tournament

1992 to Today – Operates Karate Universe in Norwalk, CT -impacting our community one black belt at a time! Karate Universe has produced over 500 black belts (1st Degree to 5th Degree)

Karate Universe

664 Main Ave.

(Townline Center Route 7)

Norwalk, CT 06851

203-849-1234

www.karateuniverse.com